INSIDE
Out

YOUR BODY IS TALKING

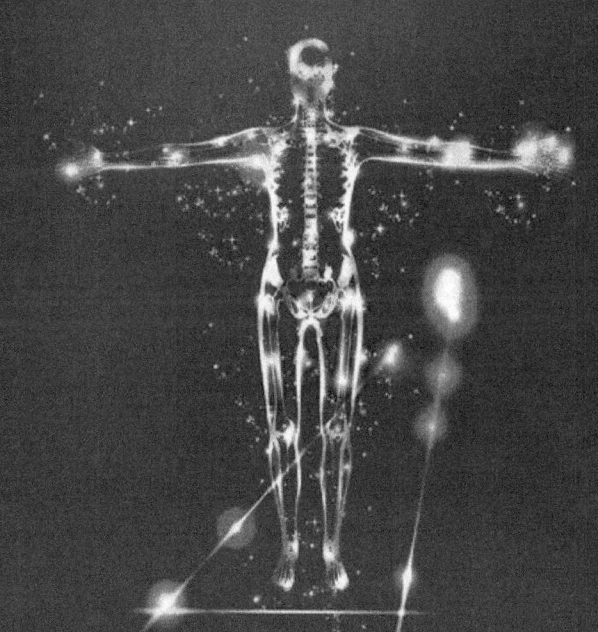

Marcia Saunders Robinson **CNHP, DE**

ISBN-13: 9781540716996

Jackson
PUBLISHING
LET THE WORDS CHANGE YOU

Acknowledgements

Thank you to my wonderful husband Rob (Butch). You have always been there for me; to love and support me throughout our 41 years of marriage. Without your encouragement and help, I would not have written this book. I love you with all of my heart!

Thank you to my children Nicole, Chris, Portia, and my daughter-in-law, Erikka. All of you have been there for me during my many, many endeavors and helped me every step of the way. Thank you Akkirah, Chris Jr., and Khylee, my grandchildren. Whenever I got tired and frustrated, all I needed was for you all to come in and I was renewed. I love you guys!!

Finally, I'd like to thank Robyn White. You helped me edit this book, advised me, and most of all, you encouraged me along the way!

Table of Contents

INTRODUCTION *1*

CHAPTER 1 THE INNER TRUTH *3*

Meet Tiffany and Joseph

Negative emotions are designed for only short time expression, long enough for you to regroup and move forward.

CHAPTER 2 YOUR EMOTIONAL AND MENTAL HEALTH *19*

Emmanuel – Perfectionism Behavior

Carmen – Daddy-less Daughter

CHAPTER 3 YOUR PHYSICAL HEALTH *WHAT SHOWS ON THE OUTSIDE?* *29*

Physical symptoms are tangible evidence of what's going on in your unconscious and conscious mind.

CHAPTER 4 YOUR HORMONAL HEALTH *WHAT IS YOUR BODY SAYING?* *39*

Hormones released by your body talks to the brain and signal your body to react.

CHAPTER 5 MOVING FORWARD *47*

What keeps you in the hurt zone?

How to be healthy despite what's happened/happening in your life.

Introduction

Wouldn't it be nice to live a life without pain? A life that is happy, full of joy and moving forward? Of course, it would. Unfortunately, life often throws us a curveball, sometimes before we even get a chance to leave our mother's womb. The emotions that we feel from the womb and even into adulthood can greatly affect our health. The things that are said to us and how we are treated can have a tremendous emotional impact on us. As you may know from experience, anything that has had an emotional impact on you can generally be recalled and in some cases re-lived down to the smallest detail. The memory of these incidents affects us emotionally, chemically, and physically.

Perhaps for you that emotional incident took place in elementary school when a teacher raised her voice at you in class and even called you lazy. Not only did that hurt your feelings but the feelings of shame and embarrassment still sting whenever you think about it or find yourself in similar situations. Regardless of how long ago that moment was for you, you still remember it and feel bad when you think about it. Whether you know it or not those difficult, and often traumatic, emotional incidents have taken a toll on your life, particularly your health.

The hurt and the pain from embarrassing experiences cause a chemical change within our bodies that can eventually lead to painful and possibly life-threatening conditions. But why? How?

As a Health and Wellness expert, I have met with many individuals with ailments, pains, and life-threatening diseases. When I took the time to listen to my clients, I discovered that many of the health issues stemmed from the emotional trauma in their lives that had not been healed. Hurtful things that were said and done early in their lives were buried deep inside of them wreaking havoc on their bodies.

If you have been struggling with health conditions and have experienced painful emotional trauma in your life, please know that you are not alone. I believe that you will find this book to be very helpful as you embark on your journey towards better health and wellness.

Some Questions this book will answer:

After years of dealing with past rejection, hurt, anger, and bitterness, you may be wondering:

1. **How do I get out of the "hurt zones" of life?**
2. **How do I keep my past from defining me and move forward?**
3. **How do I learn to love myself?**

CHAPTER 1

The Inner Truth

Tiffany's Story:

When Tiffany met me, she was 45 years old, sick and depressed. She was just diagnosed with diabetes. Recently, her grandmother died from complications from diabetes, so she was alarmed and worried about her own diagnosis. After a few sessions, she realized that most of her health issues stemmed from emotional trauma she suffered in her youth. The truth is Tiffany's story is not much different than your story. Life is hard especially if you do not take the proper steps to heal your inner child. A look at Tiffany's story will show not only how trials and tribulations can make you sick, but also how addressing their root cause will make you whole and well again.

Tiffany's story:

My mom was an 18-year-old high school senior when I was born. When she found out that she was pregnant, she knew that abortion was not an option. Therefore, she had to start thinking about how she was going to take care of me. Unfortunately, my dad wasn't much help. He was a sophomore in college and wasn't interested in interrupting his studies to take care of the consequences of a summer fling. He had dreams of becoming an engineer and a baby would derail his whole plan. Needless to say, it didn't take long for him to stop calling my mom or to stop returning her calls.

Fortunately, my mother and I weren't completely alone. My grandmother was our saving grace. She had my mother at 16 and was also abandoned by her baby's father, so she knew how hard it was going to be for my mom as a single teenage mother. I found solace in my grandmother. When my mom's resentment towards my father began to be directed towards me, she comforted me. My grandmother was the one constant source of love in my life. Unfortunately, her love for me only made my mother jealous. She would always argue with my grandmother about how nice she was treating me and how my grandmother was never that nice to her when she was growing up. It seemed like the closer I became with my grandmother, the farther my mom and I grew apart.

Living with my mother's jealousy and hatred for my father was awful. My mom always told me how much I looked like my father. I had his round eyes, his mouth, and small ears. To her dismay, I was left with her big nose and nappy hair. Whenever she reminded me that I looked or acted like my father, her voice dripped with disgust. I was a constant reminder of the man who left her to raise their child alone. In fact, according to her, I was the reason why she didn't go to college or have a great job. I ruined her life.

When life at home with my mother became rough, I would lie in my bed and daydream about what life would be like if I lived with my dad. By the time I was in middle school, I heard that he had graduated college and had even found himself a good job. I prayed every night that he would come pick me up and ask me to live with him. The truth was I couldn't even get him to call me back. I always felt so alone when there were father-daughter dances at school. All of the other girls would be so excited to dance with their dads and mine didn't even know my favorite color. I spent night after night trying to figure out what was so wrong with me that my own father didn't love me enough to call me or to spend time with me. It wasn't until much later in life that I realized how deeply being a daddy-less daughter affected me.

Despite my troubles at home, I was a really good student. I made straight A's, was a part of the school choir, Student Council, the debate team, you name it! Yet, and still, nothing I did was good enough for my mother. By the time I was a sophomore in high school, I stopped trying so hard. At this point, I had developed quite a curvy body and became rather popular with the guys at school. I loved the attention they gave me. Eventually, my shirts got tighter, skirts got shorter and the attention kept on coming. I wasn't used to this kind of attention. I never really felt pretty before. My father didn't love me; my mom always said I was ugly, and I never quite believed my grandma when she said I was beautiful every Sunday morning on our way to church. I felt like she was just saying that because I was her granddaughter. The kind of attention that I received from the boys at school was something that I didn't know I wanted until I actually had it. Eventually, I began to have sex with a few guys. I quickly realized that they were just hanging out with me to get what they *really* wanted, and then they'd leave. Even though I was popular with the guys, I never had a steady boyfriend. A small part of me couldn't really blame them. I mean my own father didn't love me so how could I expect them to love me?

My popularity with the boys gave me quite a few female enemies at school. They called me every name in the book. I was a slut, whore, hoe, tramp, etc. Though it hurt not to have any girlfriends, I convinced myself that they were just jealous that all of the boys liked me and not them. By the time I turned 17, I became pregnant. I had been having sex with so many boys that I had no clue who the father was. I thought the father might be this one guy named Joseph, but I wasn't completely sure. Even still, I told Joseph that it was his baby and after a lot of convincing on my part, he accepted responsibility. I was surprised but happy. I was finally going to have a family of my own.

Six weeks before I graduated from high school, I gave birth to my daughter Andrea. Joseph and I both graduated from high school and decided to move in together to raise our daughter. He found a job at a warehouse and I worked part-time at a hair salon and attended a local community college. My grandmother looked after the baby. After a few years, I graduated from college. Joseph and I got married and things seemed to be looking up for us. Everything was going well until I found out that Joseph was cheating on me. I couldn't believe it. After all that I had given him, I never thought that he'd betray me. He ended up apologizing, promised that he wouldn't do it again and that he'd stop seeing the other woman. He never kept any of those promises.

I thought that if I changed the way I dressed or had more kids he'd change and love me again, but it didn't work. After years of being cheated on and feeling like I wasn't enough, I finally packed my kids up and left Joseph. I was now on my own and found myself living in Section 8 housing, struggling to feed my kids with the little bit of food stamps I received. After some months, I got back on my feet and managed to get a job as a Management Analyst making pretty good money. My kids were adjusting, and I enjoyed my job. Life was turning itself around until I went for a routine physical. It was then that my doctor diagnosed me with diabetes, high blood pressure, and high cholesterol. I was devastated. How could I let this happen to me? At 45, I felt like I was way too young to be dealing with these kinds of illnesses and diseases. But I was, and I had no idea how to fix it. Soon after my diagnosis, a friend of mine connected me with Marcia. I was nervous about seeing her, but I'm so glad that I did.

After meeting with me and listening to my story, Marcia realized that my tumultuous childhood and young adult years actually played a huge role in my sickness. I had no idea that having a difficult childhood could impact my health. She helped me reconcile with my past, understand how those negative emotions were wreaking havoc on my body and helped me to move forward with my life. Thanks to her guidance and advice I have worked hard to release my anger towards my mother, my bitterness towards my father, and my hatred for my ex-husband. After I cleared my mind and emotions, I started taking better care of my body. Soon, my diabetes, high blood pressure, and high cholesterol were all under control. With a clean slate, I've been able to discover my passion and open up my dream business- a bakery! I even remarried. I feel like I've gotten my life back, and I'm so thankful."

Like most people, Tiffany had no idea that emotional trauma affects the body physically, mentally, and even chemically. She felt as though her condition had snuck up on her, but the truth is all of the stress and trauma in her life created the perfect environment for sickness to grow. Oftentimes, you have no idea how much you are holding yourself back until you take the time to free yourself. You deserve so much more out of life and owe it to yourself to listen to your body. Listen to it carefully as it tends to speak from the inside out.

Tiffany's husband, Joseph, also learned to listen to his body after his world came crumbling down around him. Though he wasn't the best husband to Tiffany, Joseph had his own set of troubles in life that probably led to his womanizing and philandering.

Joseph's story:

One of my earliest memories of my mother is an early Sunday morning just before church. I had to be around five or six- years old. On this bright and sunny morning, my mom was getting my twin sister and I ready for church. I had picked out one of my favorite outfits that I got from my grandpa; it was a light gray suit with a light peachy colored shirt, and matching gray vest. I was so excited to wear it that I hurried to dress myself and went to show my mother. I figured she'd be proud of me for dressing myself and picking out a nice Sunday outfit. Instead, she burst out laughing and told me that I was way too dark to wear that color shirt. She kept telling me that I was black as night, and that shirt made me look like a fool. That was the first time that I ever felt like I hated my skin. My mom had a caramel brown complexion like my sister, but I had a deep, dark chocolate brown complexion like my father and my grandpa (my mom's father). Even though I looked just like her dad and my father, the love of her life, my mother's words made me feel like the ugliest kid she'd ever seen.

After she laughed at me, I remember running to my dad and crying while I told him what happened. He smiled, hugged me, and told me that he used to get teased about his skin too and that the best men in his family had the same skin as I did and that it was nothing to be ashamed of. Though his reassurances made me feel better, that feeling was only temporary. Ever since that day, I've always been self-conscious about my skin. It got so bad that I hated taking pictures. My mom would have to force me to participate in the annual family pictures. I would even try to skip picture day at school. No matter what was happening in the picture, all I could see was my super dark skin and how much darker I was than everyone else. It didn't help that my mom and sister would tease me and say things like "good thing we took pictures during the day time or else we wouldn't be able to see Joey at all!" I would laugh it off, but deep down inside it hurt.

The kids at school were no better. They'd call me black bean, tar baby, blacky, and everything that made being black bad! At first it would make me cry, but then I started getting mad and I'd start fighting the kids who teased me. By the time I got to middle school, my anger was out of control. By 7th grade, my dad had gotten tired of me acting out in school and decided to take me to the local boxing club. When we walked in he said, "Son, I get why you're angry but you can't keep fighting in school. The only place you can fight is here in this club, so take all of that pain and that anger and leave it in the ring." So I did, and boxing soon became our new ritual. Almost every afternoon after school, he'd take me to the boxing club and he'd coach me. I learned how to punch properly, jab, duck, and even got to spar with some of the other kids who were training. I got my butt kicked several times, but it felt good to release all of that anger and sadness. We went so often that I actually got pretty good at boxing and started competing with other kids my age.

By the time I reached high school, I was ranking regionally as a youth boxer with hopes of reaching the state finals. All of those dreams came crashing down when my dad got killed in a car accident. We were on the way home from the boxing club when a drunk driver swerved and hit us head-on. I was pretty banged up with both a broken arm and leg, but dad wasn't so lucky. His injuries were so bad that he never made it through surgery. I was in 9th grade and never felt so lost in my life. My dad was my best friend, and now suddenly he was gone. I was stuck in a house with a mom who unmercifully teased me, and with a sister who was deep in her own world and didn't seem to even think about me. After dad passed, I stopped going to the boxing club. The thought of being there without him hurt way too much, so I started hanging with some kids from the neighborhood. Before I knew it, I was back to fighting in school and now hustling drugs in the streets. That's when the girls started to notice me. I had the fresh clothes, nice ride, and plenty of money, so the girls started to pay me more attention. This was the first time that I didn't feel like the ugliest person in the room. Despite my dark skin, girls flocked to me and I loved that feeling. This one girl, Tiffany, was so fine. I couldn't believe that she actually wanted to talk to me. She was sexy with her low cut shirts, tight jeans, and word on the street was she'd give it up if you played your cards right, and I was definitely trying to get into that. We started hanging out, and eventually we were having sex on the regular. She was honestly the first girl that made me feel wanted and desired. Everything was good until I found out that I wasn't the only one she was kickin' it with, and on top of that she was pregnant. After I found out she was sleeping around on me, I didn't want anything to do with her. She convinced me that it was my kid, so I couldn't leave. I knew what it was like to grow up with my dad, and I wanted to be that same kind of father to my kid that my dad was to me.

Six weeks before graduation, our baby girl, Andrea was born. At that moment, I felt closer to my dad. Holding my newborn daughter made me realize that I was feeling what my dad was feeling when my sister and I were born. It was true, unconditional love, and I needed a lot of that in my life. Andrea made me so happy. Even though I didn't get a chance to go to college or to keep pursuing my boxing career, I didn't mind getting a job at the local warehouse because I was doing it to take care of my daughter. I'd do anything for her. Right after Andrea was born, Tiffany and I decided to move in together. I was still hustling in the streets when I wasn't at the warehouse, and Tiff worked at a hair salon and went to school part-time.

I'd be lying if I said that I didn't resent the fact that Tiff got a chance to follow her dreams, and I didn't. Truth be told, I really missed boxing, and when I found out that Tiff was pregnant, I made it a point to get back into the ring and to start training again. I just knew that if I could make it to nationals or even the Olympics that we'd be set, and my baby girl wouldn't have to want for a thing. I got scouted by a few major boxing leagues in New York and Los Angeles, but I couldn't leave my daughter behind, so I stayed with Tiffany and got a job. I was hoping that I'd pick boxing back up once Tiff finished school. Before we knew it, we had two more kids and boxing just wasn't going to happen anymore. Just knowing that I'd never be the next boxing champ really made my blood boil.

Since boxing was no longer in the picture, I went back to what used to make me feel good. I worked, hung out with my guys, and sought the attention of other women. Don't get me wrong, over the years, I grew to love Tiffany. She was beautiful, smart, and took great care of our kids. But she didn't look at me the way she used to when we were kids. She got so caught up in taking care of the kids and work that she didn't seem to care about me anymore. The further away we got from each other, the more I started to feel like she wasn't attracted to me anymore. Did she finally see what my mother saw? Was I now just an ugly black guy? Did she still think that I was sexy? The self-doubt began to sink into my skin. The more they sunk in, the more I thought Tiffany saw me as being needy, dark and stupid. She never said it, but this is what I thought.

To erase my doubts, I started spending time with this girl I knew from the bank named Cara. Every Friday, I'd go cash my check and see Cara. The first time I saw Cara, I told her she had pretty eyes. She gave me a wide smile and began taking extra time to chat with me when I came to her window. She made me feel wanted, so I asked her out to dinner one night. She said yes. During dinner, Cara told me how she looked forward to seeing me on Fridays. I felt good about myself that night, and I didn't want it to end, so I made sure that it didn't. That night was the beginning of my affair with Cara. Cara had her own rejection issues. At night, she would go home alone from work and sometimes drink a whole bottle of wine and smoke weed to escape the pain and loneliness she felt. She had a beautiful smile but was not very attractive, and I could see right away that when I gave her a compliment it made her heart leap. When I was with Cara, I felt like I was somebody. I loved Tiffany, and she would tell me I looked good, but I always doubted that she really meant it. I needed the praise and affirmation of others, and Cara supplied that for me. This was my "other life" that Cara and I were living, and I thought I was hiding it pretty good until it blew up in my face.

When Tiffany confronted me about the text messages she saw from Cara, I saw the hurt in Tiffany's eyes. I felt so bad. How could I do this to her? She's my wife; the mother of my kids. I'm supposed to protect her and not to betray her. But I couldn't explain exactly why another woman enticed me so much. Honestly, I could have explained my feelings to her, but I thought she'd see me as weak. I couldn't have my wife thinking that I was weak and lacked confidence (even if I really did). What hurt me the most was knowing that my dad would be disappointed in me. I apologized to her over and over and even promised that I'd end the affair.

It was hard, but I ended it with Cara. I even started going to a different branch of the bank to avoid seeing her, but I honestly missed how I felt about myself when I was with her. Although the kids were amazing and Tiffany thanked me for helping her and for the things I did at home, I just didn't feel needed like I did with Cara. Tiffany was smart and together, unlike Cara whose life was a mess. If I didn't feel like having sex with Tiffany, she'd accuse me of cheating even though there wasn't any proof. It's like Tiffany and I were speaking two different languages. I couldn't take it anymore, so I called Cara and met her for breakfast one Saturday morning. Our second affair started that morning over coffee and eggs, and I no longer felt bad. Although I was leading a double life, I felt I deserved this! I worked 50 plus hours a week, kept a roof over our heads, and never missed a game or recital. I deserved to be happy too! I deserved to feel loved and needed. To soothe my guilty feelings, I told myself that Tiffany didn't really love me. All she really wanted was my paycheck. Cara made me feel important. Cara needed me. She made me feel like a man, and I wasn't letting that go again.

This went on for almost a year until I started experiencing some embarrassing health issues. No matter what I did, I struggled with erectile dysfunction. Viagra didn't work. Porn didn't work. Nothing worked! At first Cara was understanding. She figured it was the stress at work or

Tiffany's nagging that was getting to me, but it never got better. One night after it happened again, Cara told me that it wasn't working for her anymore and felt we should see different people. I was stunned. I couldn't believe it. I was so angry; I punched a hole in her wall before I left. I felt like I had been punched in the gut. All I could think, "Damn, mama was right. Maybe no one *will* ever want me." I went home feeling so rejected that when Tiffany asked me where I had been, I lost it. I yelled and screamed at her. I called her awful names that I soon regretted. I felt awful. I went downstairs to be alone to escape my misery by looking at television or rather to let the television watch me while I indulged in self-pity. I felt like Tiffany had officially taken away my dreams of becoming a pro boxer, and now Cara had rejected me after all I had done for her!!

The next morning, I woke up to an empty house. My kids were gone; Tiffany's side of the closet was bare, and the car was gone. She had left me. I tried calling her, but my calls went straight to voicemail. What had I done?! Would I ever see my kids again? I called Tiffany every single day for 6 months. After that, I just gave up. I had ruined my own life and now had nothing left. Then one day, I got a call from a woman named Marcia. She had been working with Tiffany as a wellness coach and had some questions for me. We agreed to meet at her office the next day to talk. Before I knew it, I was in her office crying like a baby. She was able to see right through my tough exterior and helped me see the true cause behind my womanizing behavior. I had no idea that my insecurity about my skin complexion caused so much stress on my body that it began to affect my sexual health. I would have never thought there was a connection between my feelings about my complexion and my inability to get an erection.

There's truly no excuse for how I treated Tiffany, but it felt great to have someone acknowledge my life struggles and to see that deep down I really wasn't a bad person. She couldn't work with me directly, and recommended that I work with another coach. He changed my life! Talking to my coach about my lifelong insecurities helped me to see the power that lies within self-love. I now understand that men need self-love and self-care too! Since working with him, I took a leap of faith and started my own boxing club. Not only do I own the club, but also I coach many young men who were just like me. My dad would be proud of how I honor and carry on his legacy. While I'm coaching my kids, I also incorporate positive affirmations before each session so they know how powerful, amazing, and loved they are. Even if they don't hear the words "I love you" from home, I make sure that they hear them from me every time they see me. I've met a wonderful woman who will be my wife next year, and I've lost over 50 pounds! I've even resolved my erectile dysfunction issue. I know it sounds crazy, but there really is a link between our unresolved issues and our health.

Hearing Joey's story always gives me goose bumps! How many of you have ever been told that you were too fat, too dark, too light, too short, too tall, too whatever to do something? At some point in your life, you have faced criticism from people. Sometimes the most hurtful criticism comes

17

from the people who are supposed to love us the most. I have worked with people who have struggled with rejection, various forms of abuse, abandonment issues, etc. The common thread between all of these issues is that more often than not, they trickle down into your health and can lead to dangerous health conditions. For Tiffany, her pain of rejection from her mom and abandonment by her dad and husband made her neglect and abandon her health. Whereas the mistreatment Joey experienced from his mother caused him to have low self-esteem and made the very organ used to exhibit his love to dysfunction. Though Joey's issue of erectile dysfunction may seem like a simple fix, sexual health issues can become very serious if not quickly and properly addressed. I say all of this to say, that the first few steps to overcoming the challenges that you have faced in your life is to acknowledge their presence and to identify how it affects all aspects of your life. In the next chapter we'll talk about how the challenges in your life have affected your thoughts and mental health.

CHAPTER 2

Your Emotional and Mental Health

We have a physical body that has an emotional and chemical component to it. It is all one and does not work independently of the other. Our personal life challenges greatly affect us mentally and emotionally. We will be talking briefly and generally about mental and emotional health. Now, I want to begin by saying that this book is in no way meant to diagnose you with any sort of disease (mental, physical or hormonal). It is simply meant to show you how certain life situations have affected some people and may help you see yourself in some of these stories. I will introduce you to Emmanuel and Carmen who will be sharing their stories with you a bit later in the chapter.

Our emotions can generally be broken down into two categories: pleasant (positive) and unpleasant (negative). Pleasant emotions include happiness, joy, love, hope, gratitude, etc. Unpleasant emotions include hate, anger, bitterness, envy, fear, anxiety, sadness, upset, unforgiveness, etc. All of these emotions are perfectly normal and are even signs of healthy emotional behavior. It is important that you know that you are not a robot. You can and will feel a mix of emotions depending on what is going on around you. Do not be afraid to feel emotions like fear, sadness, or anger. They may be uncomfortable in the moment, but they serve a purpose and can even keep you safe from danger.

In fact, scientists have discovered unpleasant emotions like fear, anger, hatred, jealousy, and sadness are actually designed to keep you safe. Fear helps your body prepare to flee from potential threats; whereas anger helps you fight off predators that may be trying to harm you in one way or another. However, these unpleasant emotions are only supposed to be short-lived. After you have run away from the threat or officially defeated the predator, those emotions of fear and anger are supposed to subside. Unfortunately, many people who have gone through traumatic emotional situations struggle to move past those unpleasant emotions.

When those unpleasant emotions become long lasting, they then can begin to breed emotions like resentment which can cause stress on the body. We will get into stress in the next chapter, but I want to emphasize how dangerous stress is to your health. Acute (short-lived) stress is a good thing. It keeps you out of danger and can be exhilarating like riding on your favorite rollercoaster or completing a marathon. However, chronic (long-lasting) stress can lead to bad habits, chronic diseases such as diabetes, heart disease, and ultimately a shorter lifespan.

Let's meet Emmanuel. His life struggles and circumstances have left him feeling overwhelmed and anxious.

Emmanuel's Story:

Hi, I'm Emmanuel. I'm 21 years old and I'm a senior at the University of Maryland where I'm studying biomedical engineering. Ever since I could remember, I've always wanted to be a scientist. I was obsessed with space, chemistry, and everything in between. At least once a month, my dad and I would go to the local science museum and I'd be amazed at all of the cool exhibits. The thing I loved about science was that it was mostly numbers which I love because I have a learning disability called dyslexia. Being dyslexic means that words and letters get scrambled which makes it harder for me to read, especially out loud. I've always struggled with reading and English classes, but my math and science classes were my refuge. Regardless of how I looked at it, 1 + 1 would always equal 2.

Math and Science classes were the only ones where I truly felt as smart as my classmates. When it came time to apply for college, I asked my English teacher if he would write me a letter of recommendation and he looked me square in the face and told me that I was not college material, and I should just think about going straight into the workforce. When I told him that I had dreams of becoming a scientist, he just laughed and told me to find a more realistic dream that I could actually accomplish. I was so hurt; I couldn't believe that a teacher would tell me something like that. I told my parents what he said, and they promised me that they would do everything they could to help me get into college, and I believed them. I worked so hard and was so proud when that University of Maryland acceptance letter came in the mail. Yet, and still that little voice in my head kept saying, "you're going to mess up if things aren't perfect" or "you've got to be perfect to show Mr. Willis that he was wrong."

Freshman year came and went. I finished my first year of college with a 3.9 GPA. I was so excited. My confidence was through the roof! Then sophomore and junior years came and the classes became harder. As the classes became harder, the less I slept. The less I slept; the more anxious I became. Until one day, I had a full blown anxiety attack in the middle of my biomedical engineering lab. I was so embarrassed. How was I supposed to be a world-famous scientist if I couldn't even make it through college?? I started to think that Mr. Willis was right. Maybe I wasn't being realistic with my dreams? Maybe I really wasn't cut out to be a scientist after all? Even though my anxiety was through the roof, I kept pushing myself. After the spring semester of my sophomore year, I started having severe pain all over my body. No matter what I did, my muscles ached and bones hurt so bad that I could barely get out of bed for class. My doctors just kept telling me they couldn't find anything wrong, and that I was just pushing myself too hard; but I couldn't afford to take time off. I had to keep going. Unfortunately, my "go, go, go" attitude just made my pain and anxiety worse.

After my third anxiety attack, I decided to book an appointment with my campus therapist/counselor. She talked to me about something called perfectionism and how it stems from feeling or being told that we weren't good enough or would never be something. I had no idea that I had internalized what Mr. Willis said to me all those years ago. I thought I was over it. I mean, I made it to college and I had great grades, but the stress of my high standards and fear of failure were crippling. At first, I really didn't take this perfectionism thing seriously. I took pride in calling myself a perfectionist. I thought it meant that I liked to have things in order and to do things in the best way. In actuality, my perfectionism caused me more harm than good. My counselor told me that people who struggle with the bad side of perfectionism often deal with depression, anxiety, and are even more likely to commit suicide. I had no idea that my unresolved hurt and pain could possibly cost me my life. In addition, perfectionists are more likely to experience extreme fatigue and even fibromyalgia which was what was causing pain all over my body. Though it was scary hearing that I was dealing with such a scary issue, it felt good to know that I wasn't imagining my pain nor was I feeling anxious without a reason. With my counselor's, help I've found ways to cope with my anxiety and I'm even having less pain. I'm more aware of my emotions and I deal with them as soon as possible to avoid internalizing them and harming my body even more than I have already. It's a hard journey, but I haven't been this happy in a very long time.

I am so happy that Emmanuel decided to share his story with me. His story is one in which many people can relate. Many want to achieve their dreams and goals so much that they will push themselves to dangerous limits to get it. Their incredibly high standards go beyond ambition and into self-destruction in the blink of an eye. Before they know it they are struggling with anxiety and feeling lost in the world, afraid to take a step in any direction for fear of failing. All of the issues that come with unresolved pain and hurt can be resolved but you have to acknowledge and identify the pain first. Setting yourself free of the hurt makes room for you to heal the many parts of your life.

Just last year I met the most amazing and loving young woman who came to me because of her struggles in her love life was spilling over into her health and work lives. Carmen came to me with the hopes of resolving her relationship issues but she ended up leaving with so much more.

Carmen's Story: **A DADDY-LESS GIRL**

When I found my coach Marcia, I was at my lowest point in my life. My seventh consecutive boyfriend was cheating on me and abruptly left me; I was overweight, suffering from an autoimmune disease, and I was feeling like a hot mess! I couldn't seem to keep a man; my relationships and friendships were in shambles. All I wanted to do was to be loved by a man, and I couldn't even do that right. So, a friend of mine suggested that I find a wellness expert and that's when Marcia entered my life. Before I met her, I went from trifling man to trifling man desperately searching for "the one." I thought my only issue was not knowing where to find him. It was obvious that the places where I met men didn't have the best quality guys. I blamed my lack of success in the love department on the guy's immaturity, selfishness, and even their inability to know a good woman when they saw one. Marcia helped me to realize that the true center of my relationship failures was my unwavering distrust of men. It wasn't until she pointed it out that I realized that she was right; I didn't trust men at all. Then, she called me out on something that rocked me to my core. She told me that my distrust of men was directly linked to me being a "daddy-less daughter." Sure, my father wasn't in my life, but I never let it bother me. Whenever he broke his promises and never showed up to any of my events, I just convinced myself that it was his loss, not mine. It sucked not having him with me during the Daddy-Daughter dances or at family day at school, but I got over it. At least I thought I was over it. The truth is that deep down inside I felt like unwanted trash. If my own father didn't think that I was worth his time then how could I expect anyone else to? I spent so many Friday evenings waiting for my dad to show up. I waited on the front porch, on stage during a recital or play, and even before prom when he promised that he'd come by and see me off. He never showed up to anything. It wasn't like he was strung out on drugs or stuck in jail. My father lived three stoplights away from me and still wouldn't come see me. In fact, he had a whole other family that he took care of and left me in the dark as if I never existed. So, in hindsight I can see why I've never been trustful of men. The first man in my life disappointed me so many times that I could not even keep count.

Working with Marcia helped me realize that my defense mechanism and choice of men were the main things that were interrupting my possibility of happiness with a man. Not only did I have a steel wall around my heart, but also I unknowingly chose men who I knew were emotionally unavailable. I created this whole system where I would choose the wrong guy, fall for them, and then be hurt and surprised when they turned out to be cheaters or bums. Little did I know that I was choosing these men because I knew that they'd never work out long term and, therefore, I wouldn't have to worry about opening up and truly trusting someone with my heart.

The stress of avoiding my emotions and dealing with stressful boyfriends led me to find comfort in food which caused me to gain over 25 pounds! Avoiding my feelings and enjoying comfort food seemed to make me happy until I started seeing my friends finding love, getting married, and having children. They all seemed so happy, and here I was bouncing from messed up relationship to messed up relationship. I couldn't get it together! Marcia helped me realize that I wouldn't find true happiness until I resolved my issues as a daddy-less daughter and learned to trust people again. She helped me see that just because my father hurt and disappointed me doesn't mean that every single man that I meet will do the same thing. It was hard to work through those issues, but once I did my life has changed for the better.

I haven't met my prince charming yet, but I've had at least one healthy relationship where I was the most vulnerable I've ever been with a man, and he stayed with me right up until we decided to call it quits. It was the most peaceful break up that I've ever experienced in my life. I do believe that I was able to dissolve that relationship because I was finally able to see the end of this relationship as just that and not another example of how I am unlovable. In addition, I started working out and finding comfort in taking care of my body rather than filling it with junk food. I feel amazing and look pretty darn good if I say so myself! You never realize just how much you're holding onto until you let it go. Marcia used an analogy that explained the damage of holding onto unresolved issues perfectly. She said that holding your arm out while holding a half full cup of water in your hand normally isn't hard. It feels lightweight and doesn't bother you one bit. But, if you have to hold that cup up for long periods of time that half full cup of water begins to feel like it weighs a ton. Your arm begins to shake, and before long you drop the cup because your muscles grown tired of holding it up for so long. That's what happens to us emotionally. When we carry around grudges from childhood bullies, unloving, absent parents, or abusive partners, holding those feelings become a heavy weight. Before we know it, your muscles are buckling without the ability to hold you up in a standing position. You begin to fall apart. It isn't until you let the pain, disappointment, and hurt go that you realize the weight of your burdens.

I am so happy that my cup of water analogy resonated with Carmen. Small pains and emotions can weigh a ton if we don't address them and let them go. As you saw with both Emmanuel and Carmen, the weight of your unresolved issues can not only cause emotional stress but also physical stress, which can cause illnesses.

In the next chapter, you will revisit the stories that you've read and see how their past struggles are directly linked to the various health issues that they experienced.

CHAPTER 3

Your Physical Health

What Shows on the Outside?

I would like to begin this discussion by first letting you know that I am not a physician and that this chapter is in no way designed for self-diagnosis nor should it replace a relationship with your primary care physician. Should you have any questions regarding the statements made in this book and how they relate to your health, please consult your physician.

Now that we have a sense of how unresolved issues can affect your mental and emotional health, let's take a look at how they can disrupt how your bodies function on a daily basis. In many cases, physical symptoms are just tangible evidence that there is something going on in your conscious and subconscious mind. Your weight issues, high blood pressure, anxiety, and sexual health issues could be indirectly related to your unresolved feelings of rejection, abandonment, self-worth, grief, and other emotional issues. Many may ask: "well, how could my blood pressure be related to my dad walking out on my mom and I when I was 9?" Well, it's not as simple as your dad left you at a young age, and now you have high blood pressure. It's more like your dad left you at a young age, and now you always have difficult relationships with men that are stressful to you. That stress causes you to overeat which has now caused you to have high blood pressure, weight gain, etc. Sometimes those bad feelings from the past are simply a catalyst which cause you to spiral out of control without you even realizing it.

Just to refresh your memory, I will summarize everyone's unresolved issue and health problem and then talk about how that issue led to the health problem. Tiffany had unresolved feelings of abandonment and low self-worth due to her father's willful absence in her life and rejection from her mother. In her 40s, Tiffany developed diabetes and high blood pressure. Her husband Joseph had unresolved issues that included grief from his father's death and lack of self-love due to constant criticism from his mother about his skin complexion. In his 40s, Joseph developed erectile dysfunction that derailed his life and confidence. Emmanuel struggled with self-confidence and self-compassion due to harsh criticism from a high school teacher. In college, Emmanuel struggled with anxiety and a pain disorder called fibromyalgia. Lastly, Carmen had unresolved feelings of abandonment and disappointment due to her absent father. Carmen struggled with weight gain and the ability to find healthy coping mechanisms.

Now, let's talk about Tiffany...

Tiffany came to me when she was newly diagnosed with both diabetes and high blood pressure. She was shocked by her diagnosis, but when I learned more about her background and current lifestyle, I wasn't so surprised. Tiffany was depressed and struggling with low self-worth which are both catalysts for chronic diseases like diabetes and high blood pressure. When you are depressed and dealing with low self-worth, you are less likely to take care of yourself. You either lack the motivation to eat well, exercise, and practice self-care or you are so busy caring for other people that you end up on the bottom of your own totem pole.

This is a situation for many women. They are either buried neck deep in past pain and hurt or are so busy keeping their families afloat that they end up with a lack of money or time to take care of themselves. In Tiffany's case, she figured that if both her father and husband couldn't love her, then what was the point of working out and doing good things for herself? She even questioned if she deserved it at all. Instead, the comfort from her pain and disappointment came in the form of food. Let's be honest, we don't call it comfort food for nothing. There's something about mac and cheese, cakes, pies, and pizza that removes all of the pain and hurt in the world. At least temporarily it makes life better. Then you wake up and feel bad about eating the whole bag of chips or gorging on half of that pound cake. That's when the negative self-talk begins. For some it sounds like, "See, this is why my dad and husband didn't love me, I have no self-control!" or "Hey girl, if you keep this up you gonna be the size of a house and then no one will definitely want you!" The cycle continues over and over again until your body begins to shut down.

In order to get blood to flow throughout a bigger and heavier body, your heart has to pump harder and faster which leads to high blood pressure. Also, your body is being flooded with so much sugar that it can't handle it and that leads to diabetes. Diabetes can be a complex disease to understand, but I believe that I have found the perfect way to explain it. Picture your cells as houses in a neighborhood and your blood is the street where the houses are located. The sugar in the cakes and pies that you eat are little packages that come to each house to help the cell function properly. The local mailman called Insulin delivers the packages (sugar) to each cell every day. Insulin rings the doorbell and the cell opens up and takes the sugar. The more cakes and pies you eat, the more often Insulin has to come and deliver the sugar. Insulin comes to your cell so often that it breaks your doorbell. Every time insulin comes to deliver sugar to the cell, the cell can't open up because the doorbell is broken. Now, the porches and front lawns of each house (cell) are full of packages (sugar) because the sugar can't get in. If the sugar doesn't get into the cell, then it will build up into the blood and cause high blood sugar aka diabetes.

Tiffany's body was so stressed with the extra weight and sugar that it couldn't function properly. Thankfully, resolving her issues and developing a self-care routine has helped her get back on track. She had to realize that she was worth the care, and that if she wasn't healthy then she wouldn't be able to take care of her family the way they needed.

Joseph...

For Joseph, the fact that he was dealing with erectile dysfunction (ED) may not seem important, but ED can be a sign of heart disease. ED is a very sensitive subject for many men and can cause stress, relationship strain, and low self-esteem. Joseph had always been teased about his skin complexion and had been taught that no one would want him because he was too dark. His father was his only sense of love and validation and when he was killed, Joseph felt like he had no where to turn when things got rough. So when he became sexually active, Joseph began building his confidence around his sex life and the affection he received from women. When he began to develop erectile dysfunction and lost an important relationship because of it, it confirmed that no one would love him because he was too dark. He couldn't provide the one thing that he thought made women love him, and so his confidence began to crumble. The thing about insecurity is that it lurks everywhere. It's always in the shadows of your mind and comes out at the most inopportune times. Insecurity makes you feel like you aren't good enough to have the job you want, relationship you want, etc. It serves as a frequent reminder of how inadequate you think you are and that adds so much stress to your life. In Joseph's case, his insecurities about his skin complexion caused him to be unfaithful and to destroy his marriage and to ultimately lead to his erectile dysfunction. Though he was attracted to Cara, the stress of having to always fight off the negative thoughts while he was with her kept him from performing sexually. Dealing with ED is embarrassing and stressful on its own and coupled with a deep insecurity made it that much more difficult for Joey to overcome. It was only when Joey began working through his issues with his mother and his insecurities about his skin complexion that he started to feel better. When he started implementing positive affirmations like: "I am good enough" and "I am in control of my destiny," he started to feel more confident. With more confidence and self-love, he was finally able to address his ED and now lives a fulfilled life. Men, you have to know that you all need self-love too!

Emmanuel...

Next, we move on to Emmanuel, the smart and inspirational young man who is an aspiring engineer. After being told by a teacher that he'd never make it to college, Emmanuel began struggling with perfectionism. It was his perfectionism that helped him make good grades and get into college. However, it was also his perfectionism that caused him to develop anxiety, depression, and even fibromyalgia. For many, perfectionism is a two-sided coin. It is the driving force that helps people strive for excellence and do well on almost anything their minds desires. On the other hand, it causes them to set extremely high standards for themselves and to develop a genuine fear of failure. In Emmanuel's case, the high standards that he set for himself were rooted in this determination to prove his old teacher wrong. He wanted to show that teacher that he was smart and could make it into and *through* college.

In doing so, he stressed himself out about exams and projects. When he made a B on a test, it wasn't good enough. When people complimented him and said that he did a "good job" his only thought was "good? Why not wonderful or amazing? Good isn't good enough." All of these thoughts added more stress, which led to him developing a serious anxiety disorder. Anxiety can be crippling; it can keep you from being around friends and doing the things that you love. Your body is basically in a constant state of worry and hyper-awareness that adds to the stress that caused the anxiety in the first place. The constant stress of high expectations mixed with poor sleep led to Emmanuel developing a disorder known as fibromyalgia. Fibromyalgia is a disorder that results in chronic, widespread pain all over the body. Stress and anxiety are known to aggravate and increase the symptoms of fibromyalgia, as experienced by Emmanuel. When he finally decided to seek the help of a counselor and started taking better care of himself, Emmanuel noticed fewer fibromyalgia flare-ups and less anxiety. By acknowledging what his high school teacher said about him and how much it hurt him, Emmanuel was able to move past it. He was finally able to reconcile with that part of his past and look forward to his bright future.

Carmen...

Lastly, Carmen is a young woman who dealt with a common issue: feeling unlovable and abandoned by her absentee father. Carmen is what I like to call a "Daddy-less daughter." She yearns for the love and affection from men, but feels she is unworthy of this love because her own father never gave it to her. How could she expect random men to love her when her own father didn't care about her? Instead of dealing with her hurt and pain, Carmen put up an impenetrable wall around her heart and subconsciously chose to date emotionally unavailable men. These stressful relationships gnawed at her self-esteem and when she felt like the pain was getting to be too much, she began to comfort herself with food. Once her body realized that eating released special chemicals called endorphins (we'll talk about those in the next chapter) that made her feel better; it craved more and more food.

When I started working with Carmen, she was 25 pounds overweight and very unhappy. Though it took a while to break through that wall around her heart, once the break occurred, Carmen was able to release all of the pain and disappointment that she had kept bottled up for so long. When you numb yourself from pain, you also numb ourselves from joy too. Carmen chose to numb herself with food and her weight gain posed a serious threat to her health. Together, we came up with a plan to help her make better food decisions, exercise, and weight lost. The most important part of that plan was helping her find alternate ways to cope with stress, disappointment, and hurt. Instead of turning to the ice cream or pizza, Carmen used yoga, adopted a prayer schedule, and even used exercise as a coping mechanism. All of these small changes yielded big results and changed her life for the better.

At some point, the pain and disappointment that you are ignoring or refusing to address will catch up with you. In some people, it will manifest in anxiety or depression while in others it will manifest as physical disease. You may think that past hurt has nothing to do with your elevated blood pressure or auto-immune disease like lupus but addressing those issues could actually be the key to easing your symptoms and effectively managing your health.

CHAPTER 4

Your Hormonal Health

What Is Your Body Saying?

In the last chapter you may have noticed that I mentioned something called endorphins and I'm pretty sure you were thinking something along the lines of "what on earth is an endorphin?" Well, endorphins are chemical signals in the brain that are released during strenuous exercise, emotional stress, and pain. These endorphins help relieve pain and cause you to feel intense pleasure and/or euphoria. Basically, endorphins are your feel good chemicals that can be triggered by many different factors. In addition to endorphins, there are many hormones that are released in the body that play a role in your health and can even be affected by emotional stress. Hormones are chemicals that are secreted by glands and used by the body to communicate between organs and tissues. They regulate your digestion, metabolism, breathing, sleep, growth, and mood to name a few. A few hormones that you might recognize or have heard of before include: estrogen, testosterone, progesterone, insulin, thyroid stimulating hormone (TSH), growth hormone, cortisol, adrenaline, oxytocin, etc. All four of my past clients had hormone disruption which either led to their disease or played some sort of role in its development. Clearing their emotional baggage and creating a healthy lifestyle gave my clients an opportunity to regulate those hormones and to get their lives back on track.

Tiffany...

In Tiffany's case, her stress and overeating lead to the disruption of two common hormones: a) insulin and b) cortisol. Insulin is a hormone that is secreted by a small organ just behind your stomach known as the pancreas. The pancreas releases insulin into the bloodstream when you've eaten a lot of carbohydrates. Insulin helps the body direct the sugar into the cells so it can be used for energy. Remember, insulin is the local mailman who delivers sugar to your cells. When your cells no longer respond to insulin, all of that sugar is left in your blood stream where it becomes type II diabetes.

When the body no longer responds to insulin, it is called insulin resistance and it is the first stage before the onset of diabetes. Insulin resistance is also a precursor to heart disease, Alzheimer's, and cancer, just to name a few diseases. Excess sugar in your blood can cause inflammation and tissue damage throughout your body.

Cortisol on the other hand is known as the stress hormone. Remember when we talked about fear being an emotion that helps you flee from danger? Well, when you feel fearful and need to run from a threat, cortisol is one of the "fight or flight" hormones that is released into your body when you are stressed. In small amounts, cortisol is helpful and even behaves as your body's natural anti-inflammatory agent. However, constant release of cortisol can do more harm than good.

Cortisol is released by two walnut-sized organs that sit right on top of our kidneys called our adrenals. When you are stressed your adrenals release cortisol into your blood which then slows down your stomach's work, increases your blood sugar, and increases your heart rate. You may be wondering why the body would feel the need to do all of this when you are stressed, but it actually makes perfect sense. Back in the days of cavemen, humans had to run away from all kinds of threats like bears and other wild animals. Cortisol is used by the body to take all of the body's energy and to use it towards running away from the threat. For example, if you need to run away from a bear your body is not going to spend its energy trying to digest your lunch, instead it is going to have your heart pump faster to push blood throughout your body (especially your brain), and it is going to have your liver push sugar into the blood so that your muscles and brain can use it to run away from the bear. The body is incredibly intelligent, and knows how to keep you safe. Unfortunately, in this world that you live in you are always stressed; your bear becomes paying bills, working at a job you, taking care of children, and coping with past hurts and pains. All of these different things bring stress into your life and stress has the power to destroy your body. In Tiffany's case, chronic stress was the reason why she leaned towards food for comfort and it also led to her developing diabetes and high blood pressure.

Joseph...

Joseph found himself struggling with a common disorder usually found in men over 40 years old, erectile dysfunction also known as ED. ED can occur due to low levels of testosterone, the male sex hormone. Testosterone is a hormone that is produced by the testes and is responsible for male reproductive development. Testosterone is also important for bone growth, sexual function, maintaining muscle mass, and a sense of well-being. As a man ages, the amount of testosterone that his body naturally makes slowly begins to decline. This decline can start as early as a man's 30s and continues throughout his life. Low levels of testosterone can also be caused by chronic illness, obesity, and stress. When a man is experiencing low levels of testosterone, he may notice a reduction in sex drive, concentration, bouts of depression, and erectile dysfunction. Though Joseph's ED was not caused solely by low testosterone, it is important for men to be aware of their testosterone levels as they age especially if they are noticing symptoms that affect their daily lives. There are also times when a man's testosterone converts into estrogen, commonly thought to be a female hormone; however, both men and women have estrogen, progesterone and testosterone, only in different amounts. The conversion of testosterone to estrogen is called aromatase. This conversion has many of the same symptoms as low testosterone. This is why men suffering from ED should speak with their physicians about having a hormonal panel blood test to determine the exact cause of their symptoms.

In addition, Joseph's condition was aggravated by the high levels of stress that he was dealing with due to his insecurities and feelings of inadequacy. Chronic stress can weaken your adrenal glands, flood your bodies with cortisol, and wreak havoc on your bodies.

Emmanuel...

Emmanuel suffered from anxiety due to high levels of stress. His struggle with perfectionism affected the following hormones: cortisol, and adrenaline. We already talked about cortisol earlier in this chapter. Stress was a central part to all of his health issues and that stress stemmed from unresolved emotional issues and poor coping skills. Another stress hormone that is often secreted with cortisol is adrenaline. Yep, the thing that makes your heart race and gives you a brief rush of pleasure after a roller coaster ride or other scary adventures. That's an adrenaline rush. Adrenaline, also known as epinephrine is a stress hormone and also a medication that is used in severe allergic reactions (ex: the EpiPen®) and during cardiac arrest (when your heart stops beating). Adrenaline increases blood flow to the muscles, heart rate and blood sugar. Every emotional response has three parts to it: 1) a behavioral component, 2) an autonomic (involuntary) component, and 3) a hormonal component. The hormonal component includes the release of cortisol and adrenaline. The most common emotions that trigger the release of these stress hormones are fear and anxiety. In Emmanuel's case, he suffered from anxiety and an overwhelming fear of failure. The excess adrenaline in his system and the stress from his incredibly high standards caused Emmanuel to suffer panic attacks. His body even developed a disease called fibromyalgia which is aggravated by both stress and anxiety.

Carmen...

Carmen's abandonment issues and stress led to her overeating and subsequent weight gain. As mentioned previously, cortisol can wreak havoc on the body and was a trigger for her weight gain. An additional hormone that played a role in Carmen's abandonment issues is oxytocin. Oxytocin is a hormone that is involved in social connections, uterine contractions during labor, and lactation during breastfeeding. In regards to social behavior, oxytocin causes an overwhelming sense of contentment, calmness and security when in the presence of a loved one. Carmen never experienced this with her father, so she craved it from other men in her life. Being in a relationship released lots of oxytocin which made Carmen feel wanted, loved, and less anxious. In addition, being in a relationship released lots of dopamine into her system. Dopamine is a chemical in the brain that triggers motivation, reinforcement, and reward. It essentially makes you feel good, so when Carmen could no longer get that good feeling from her boyfriends, she turned to food. It was important for Carmen to find other ways to release dopamine and feel good without the help of food. This is where self-care and good coping skills came in handy.

Hormones can be a complicated topic, and I hope this chapter helped to clarify the importance of hormones and how emotional stress (and stress in general) affect your body's response to hormones. Rather than think of hormones like cortisol as the bad guy, think of it as a tool that is very useful but under the wrong conditions it causes a lot of harm. This is why staying healthy and taking care of yourself should be a top priority.

CHAPTER 5

Moving Forward

The first thing that you will have to realize is that the Storms of Life are going to be ever present during your lifetime. Unfortunately, you cannot have a life without bad times. Fortunately, you can look at these bad times as moments of growth and reasons to appreciate the good times you experience.

Even though the storms of life will always be present, you can move forward from past hurt and learn how to handle future pain and disappointment.

It is important to recognize that many of the common illnesses you have are directly related to how you have chosen to handle negative things that happen. Whether it's rejection from a parent or spouse, being fired from a job, betrayed by your best friend, illness, or death, holding on to or suppressing negative emotions is keeping you from moving forward. Many of you are standing in quicksand, and stuck in how you have viewed your circumstances, and in how you see yourself as a result of your decisions. Now, it's time to move forward, but you are stuck in not knowing how to do it.

How to move forward?

Life is like a computer. Sometimes your computer will get bogged down by lots and lots of old files running and cause slow processing. In order for it to run faster and more efficiently, you have to go in and clean out your history file. This cleans out the old junk and allows space for new information. This allows your computers to work faster and more efficiently so you can get more work done.

Your mind is your computer. If you constantly keep years and years of hurt and anger to accumulate in your mind and heart, like the computer, you will slow down internally. Your hormones and internal chemistry become imbalanced, and you get sick. When this happens to you as a woman, it causes fibroids, hot flashes, and mood swings. For men, you develop erectile dysfunction and big bellies. Stress and hormone imbalance increase your chances of developing lupus, cancer, diabetes, high blood pressure, becoming depressed and ultimately your inability to move forward.

6 Steps to take to move forward with your life...

1. **Let go of negative people** – When you leave a conversation with a person you should feel good about yourself. That interaction should be encouraging and uplifting. If you leave conversations and interactions feeling bad about yourself and your life, then you need to free yourself from them. Spend your time with people who are spiritually centered, positive, healthy and likeminded. Relationships should help you, not hurt you. Surround yourself

with people who reflect the person that you want to be. Your friends should be people who you are proud to know, people you admire, who love and respect you. Your friends should be people who make your day a little brighter simply by being in it. Life is too short to spend time with people who suck the joy and peace out of you. When you free yourself from negative people, you free yourself to be YOU! Being YOU is the only HEALTHY way to truly live.

2. **Let go of those who are already gone** – The truth of the matter is that there are some people who will only be there for you as long as you have something they need. When you no longer serve a purpose to them, they will leave. By being the emotionally healthy person you strive to be, you will see these people for who they really are and weed these people out of your life. In the end, you will be left with some great people who you can count on. You rarely lose friends and perhaps "loved ones" who genuinely care about you. So, when people walk away from you, let them go. Your destiny is never tied to anyone who leaves you. It doesn't mean that they are bad people; it just means that their part in your story is over.

3. **Stop comparing yourself to others** – There is an old saying: "comparison is the thief of joy." It truly does rob you of joy and peace. God allows circumstances to happen in your life in order to prepare you for your future. To look at someone else and wish you had their life, doing what they are doing, or have what they

have is like wishing you had someone else's fingerprint. Just as each person's fingerprint is unique, each one of you has a unique story that is preparing you for your future. Life is an individual journey, and its one that should be lived in the best way possible. You can only live your life, not someone else's. Embrace your journey and live your best life!!

4. **Show everyone kindness and respect** – Treat everyone with kindness and respect, even those who are rude to you, not because they are nice, but because you are. There are no boundaries or classes that define a group of people who deserve to be respected. Treat everyone with the same level of respect you would give an elder and the same level of patience you would have with a baby. People will notice your kindness and blessings will come into your life because of it.

5. **Be your imperfectly perfect self** – We live in an age when everyone is trying to make you feel like you need to be like everyone else. Being emotionally healthy, you have the courage to stand up to be your awesome self! Be yourself, different from everyone else. Who appointed anyone judge and jury to say what's normal and what's not? What's normal? What's right for you may be wrong for someone else and that's okay. Dare to be different. Everyone has a different story and each story deserves to be shared. Spend more time with those who make you smile and less time with those who you feel pressured to impress. Be your imperfectly perfect self. Remember, the bible says that you

are fearfully and wonderfully made! (Psalms 139:14)

6. **Forgive people and move forward** – The bible also tells us not to be get caught in the rut of how people hold on to grudges and hurts but to be transformed by having our mind renewed so that we can move forward and get all the blessings that God has in store for us. (Romans 12:2)

Don't live your life with hate in your heart. You will end up hurting yourself more than the people you hate. Forgiveness is not saying, "What you did to me is okay." It is saying, "I'm not going to let what you did to me ruin my joy and peace." Forgiveness is the remedy. It doesn't mean you're erasing the past, or forgetting what happened. It means that you're letting go of the resentment, pain, anger, and bitterness. Instead, you are choosing to learn from the incident and move forward with your life. Remember, the less time you spend hating people who hurt you, the more time you'll have to love yourself and to love the people who love you.

Lesson on the damage that hate can have on a person:

One afternoon, a kindergarten teacher decided to play a game with her class. The teacher told each child in the class to go home and to fill a bag with some potatoes. She told the students to name each potato after a person that the child hates. So, the number of potatoes that a child put into his or her bag depended on the number of people he or she hated.

So when the day came, every child brought some potatoes with the name of the people he or she hated. Some had two potatoes; some had three while some students had up to five potatoes. The teacher then told the children to carry the potatoes in the bag with them wherever they went for one week. Days passed and the children started to complain due to the unpleasant smell of the rotten potatoes. In addition, those who had five potatoes found that the bags were really heavy and hard to carry. After one week, the children were relieved because the game finally ended.

After the game was over the teacher asked: "How did you feel while carrying the potatoes with you for one week?" The children let out their frustrations and started complaining of the trouble they experienced carrying the heavy and smelly potatoes wherever they went.

Then the teacher told them: "This is exactly the situation when you carry hatred and unforgiveness for somebody inside your heart. The stench of hatred and unforgiveness will contaminate your heart and you will carry it with you wherever you go. If you cannot tolerate the smell of rotten potatoes for just one week, can you imagine what is it like to have the stench of hatred and unforgiveness in your heart for your lifetime?"

Moral of the story: Throw away hatred and unforgiveness , so that you will not carry the burden for a lifetime. Unforgiveness harms you more than the other person!

Healthy Rules to Live By:

- **Give what you want to receive** – Don't expect what you are not willing to give. Start practicing the golden rule in all areas of your life. If you want love, give love. If you want friends, be a friend to others. If you want money, provide value. It works. It may seem hard to believe, but it really is this simple.

- **Allow others to make their own decisions** – Do not judge others from your own past experiences. They are living a different life than you are. What might be good for one person may not be good for another. What might be bad for one person might change another person's life for the better. Allow people to make their own mistakes and their own decisions. All you can do is be there for them in the good times and in the bad.

- **Pay attention to the relationship with yourself** – The relationship that you have with yourself is the most important relationship you will ever have in your lifetime. One of the most painful things in life is losing yourself in the process of loving others and forgetting that YOU are special. When was the last time someone told you that they loved you just the way you are or told you that what you think and how you feel matters? When was the last time that you thought about what you love and your purpose? When was the last time someone told you that you did a good job, or took you someplace nice simply because they know you feel happy when you're there? When was the last time that "someone" was YOU?

Though moving forward in life can be difficult it will give you peace, joy, self-love and love for others. Moving forward will free you from the quicksand you've been stuck in while continuously looking back and living in past hurts, anger, and bitterness. Moving forward will help you be the healthy person you were created to be. Taking these steps, moving forward with your life, and living in your true purpose will help you be healthy from the inside out.

Contact The Author

Marcia Saunders Robinson

insideouthebody@gmail.com

Order Book :

Inside Out

Your Body Is Talking

www.insideoutthebody.com

(301)744-7163